Falling Asleep
and
Staying Asleep

Pamela Ryan

Trafford rev.   01/31/2014

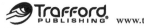 www.trafford.com

North America & international
toll-free: 1 888 232 4444 (USA & Canada)
fax: 812 355 4082

Contents

Introduction

Why is it so hard to fall asleep?

Billions of dollars are spent each year on over the counter drugs, self medication, and prescription drugs. More than one third of the U.S. population complains of always being tired.

Does your insomnia manifest itself as difficulty in falling asleep? Do you wake up soon after falling asleep? Do you take short naps to make up for your lack of sleep at night? If you are sleeping lightly and never entering the delta wave or restorative sleep stage, you may be heading for serious health problems.

Our bodies need to sleep for the whole night or at least eight hours.

You know you have insomnia when your mental state is portrayed by an inability to fall asleep or stay asleep.

After many years of trying to find ways to overcome my insomnia, this book was created as a way to share some solutions on how to defeat your sleep disorder.

If you are serious in your efforts to get needed sleep, it may require you to change your sleep patterns and certain habits.

I know the typical type "A" personality, always moving as fast as you can. When one project is finished the next one is started.

You feel like a bundle of energy. Sleeping takes time out of your busy schedule. It probably makes you mad your body needs to sleep. You feel like you have so much to do, but not enough hours in the day . . .

You know you are having problems sleeping when you begin to deny yourself enough sleep. Then you begin to use stimulants like lots of coffee, energy drinks, and any other over the counter remedies to help you stay awake.

If you are averaging only 4-6 hours of sleep a night and continue taking all the stimulants you pump into your body, it will not take long before your body and mind become dysfunctional and disoriented. Your body needs that deep delta wave sleep that restores and repairs your cells. When you neglect your body's need for sleep, it will take its toll on you unexpectedly.

After you decide to change some of your bad habits and take charge of your sleep, you will understand how you can tap into the amazing energy our bodies consume and produce daily. The solution is to get into harmony with your *body, mind, and spirit.*

Chapter 1

Checklist

The need for Comfort is paramount for getting the good night sleep you crave. For starters, something as simple as being in the right place, like your own bedroom will give you the edge. You know how it feels to be in your own home in your own bedroom and in your own bed, because when you are away from it you yearn for it.

Some of us will find a spot on the sofa, because we can watch the big screen TV. Then in the morning your neck hurts you have a stiff back and you haven't slept well at all.

The bedroom is a place that must invite you to sleep. It is our private place, where we can cry alone and pray alone or just be alone, or not. It must be set apart from the rest of the home.

The desire to watch TV in bed, before you try to sleep is a big mistake as it stimulates the senses. Our mind can't tell the difference between the entertainment we see on TV or the real thing. Adrenalin begins to pump through our veins and anticipation, intensity and the fight or flight reaction will keep you awake for hours after the TV program has ended. When this happens you can try to sleep and just toss and turn for hours in bed, while your brain overrides your efforts to fall asleep.

If you decide you need less sleep and then make the decision to stop fighting it, it may help you sleep later. Sleeping less means you have more time on your hands. In the past you would be trying to fall asleep, because you felt tired. Now you have the time to create the bedroom setting that you would feel comfortable to sleep in and/or stay awake in.

First and foremost and let it be said, right here right now, the mattress you have purchased to sleep on is vitally important in your quest for a good nights sleep.

Statistically, people will keep the same mattress for more than ten and up to twenty years.

Yes, it's true, we tend to overlook the importance of the mattress we will be sleeping on when we buy it, but we do.

The mattress you choose should not be purchased in haste. Think about it . . . It is on your mattress that you spend more than half your life lying down. Decisions made according to cost should be avoided.

Shopping for the new mattress in an effort to find out what your preference is, should be an adventure. Don't be shy you must test the mattress before you buy.

Do you like it firm, soft, pillow top or a temperpedic mattress?

If you share a bed with a partner you may not share preferences about the firmness, softness, or price of the mattress. There are two ways to produce a solution, the right way, and the wrong way. Kept in mind the solution is all about you getting a good night sleep.

If your partner snores, sweats a lot, tosses, and turns because they can't sleep and wakes you up, you can be sure their sleeping problem has become yours as well. The problem is not the partner, but possibly their sleeping habits that's keeping you awake.

There are beds on the market that you and your partner can control the firmness separately. Unless you choose to sleep in separate beds, try to figure it out.

You would be surprised to learn that people live with these simple solvable issues every day and even though there are easy solutions, they would rather live with the problem and continue to complain about it.

First step is to do what ever it takes, so you can get your needed sleep. If the problem is snoring and it's keeping you from a good night sleep, don't be shy, tell him/her. If the problem is incessant snoring, this happens to be a common sign of obstructive sleep apnea. With a breathing disorder that occurs during the sleep cycle, you actuality stop breathing repeatedly or it will cause an interruption of breathing. There are risks if you have developed sleep apnea, so it is important to see your physician.

Otherwise, there are dozens of product solutions for snoring on the market you can buy over the counter in any drug store. After these simple solutions, you could shop together and have fun with this.

Testing different mattresses in a furniture store, may feel weird at first. Laying down on a variety of mattresses in the store will definitely help you to make a better decision.

Your choices depend on whether or not you try out the difference between a pillow top and temperpedic mattress. After testing different types, buy the best mattress you can afford. Shop around, including online websites to find the best price. Now, lying in my new bed awake or asleep is a pleasure. Still, sleeping is always the goal . . .

Are You Blocked

Since the discovery of quantum theory, we have learned that everything is energy. Our body is made up of billions of atoms in motion that produce a frequency. These atoms are so small and moving at such a fast pace we see each other only in a solid form.

The energy they use and produce is the electrical system that runs our body, mind, and spirit, our waking and sleeping life.

Since we are made up of more than just a physical body, this book will introduce you to your power energy centers, called chakras.

The chakras produce a network of high energy centers that store power for use by our *body, mind and spirit.* Each chakra is designated with a different function and purpose. Here is the stored energy that is distributed to do various tasks (all run by our subconscious mind) through-out our body.

Energy, used or unused during the day, has a profound effect on how we sleep at night. This book will help you determine if the main culprit for your sleep disorder is excess energy that is trapped in these energy centers.

Why is energy trapped in the body?

Stress is one of the most common reasons for the lack of sleep, but the number one cause that energy gets blocked is; the lack of physical exercise. That is not the only reason. In this book we will look at some of the other causes for energy stagnation and blockages.

It is true, in the twenty first century with all our advanced knowledge of how the body works; our baby boomer generation has become overweight and lethargic. Exercise is a necessity, but where's the energy when you need it? Stored in our chakras!

We have to utilize this unused leftover energy to lead a healthy lifestyle and get our needed sleep. In other countries, their aging society practice, in public together, different forms of exercise to release these blockages.

We use a tremendous amount of energy every day in running our bodily functions that we take for granted, but that keeps us alive.

When we engage in physical exercise we burn some of the energy that is stored in our chakras. Daily exercise can use a lot of this energy, but not all energy is used to run the body's systems.

There is also energy stored in the chakras for our mental, emotional, and spiritual use. When energy is blocked here, more than physical exercise is needed to convert this negative energy.

During our journey through life we can't help but accumulate, by choice or not, negative energy. This kind of energy makes you feel tired, but you cannot fall asleep.

The information in this book is primarily addressing the way energy is stored for our body, mind, & spirit that can keep us from sleeping.

The fact that we need to sleep every night is a fascinating function of the human body that none of us can deny. Sleeping is a necessity to our mental and physical survival. Our bodies live by a twenty four hour cycle. This is called our biological clock or our **circadian rhythm.**

The sleep/wake cycle is controlled by the circadian rhythm. If you cannot get to sleep when the lights go out and the sun goes down, you can be sure that your circadian rhythm is out of sync.

It will take practice to find your body's rhythm again.

Naturally, when we are in harmony with our body, we will fall asleep according to this rhythm, without much effort. On the other hand, an energy blockage will throw off our rhythm and no matter what we do we can't fall asleep.

The blocked energy that may be a cause of your insomnia will clear with the consistent practice of the cleansing rituals found in this book, if used for 30 days. For some of us, it takes practice to do the necessary work to fall asleep.

This book describes the methods I found useful to balance the body's energy centers. The purpose is so you can fall asleep and stay asleep for a full nights rest. It takes work to first recognize and then release this blocked energy.

The exercises in this book in the form of rituals will help you recall them easily with little practice. The amount of effort it takes to understand and to use these techniques will be your ultimate gain resulting in a good night sleep.

The use of rituals and the evidence of releasing the blocked energy from our energy centers are unique in this book. Just some practical advice from a former insomniac that might help you gets your needed sleep.

Are you Hungry?

Dieting and sleeping are like a bad marriage, you may have to decide to give up one and eat your way to a good night sleep.

If you are hungry and try to sleep on an empty stomach you might as well drink a bottle of red bull.

Hunger will keep you awake while your body undergoes a natural response. The brain is notified that your body is hungry. In response, hormones are released into the blood stream. Don't go to bed hungry. With food in your stomach to digest, your body will work at digestion and not alarm your brain about your hunger.

If you're hungry, the remedy to get your needed sleep is simple, just eat something, but why not eat something that will help you sleep.

Carbohydrate rich foods that increase the concentration of **tryptophan** will have a calming effect on the body. When foods are consumed that contain tryptophan, the tryptophan is converted in the process of metabolism to **serotonin.**

Vitamin B6, pyridoxine, taken at night before you go to bed, is called the "mood vitamin" because it helps our brains **convert the amino acid L-tryptophan into a neurotransmitter** called serotonin.

Serotonin is a chemical that is important to our brain function, because it not only regulates our moods, but our sleep.

Serotonin is a neurotransmitter made in the brain. It is *not found* in foods.

A neurotransmitter is a chemical messenger that carries signals between the neurons (nerve cells) and the cells of the body. It is released into the bloodstream, specifically to help your body regulate the function of the sleep cycle, mood, anger, appetite, sexuality, and several other processes. Without neurotransmitters the brain could not tell the heart to beat, the stomach to digest, or the body to sleep!

Choose foods with tryptophan that cause **serotonin** to be released like a bowl of cereal, brown rice, a baked potato, or pasta. Tryptophan is also found in foods such as chocolate, turkey, soy products, peanuts, almonds, bananas, cabbage, broccoli, spinach, beets, oats, tomatoes, some meat, fish, chicken, and especially turkey.

Herbal sources of tryptophan are huang-gin, St. John's wort, mustard seeds, wolf berry, fenugreek, sunflower seeds, fennel, alfalfa, green cardamom, flax, anise, coriander, poppy, milk thistle, tart cherry fruit, red radish root tuber, pumpkin, watermelon, spirulina, tofu, and beans.

These foods help with serotonin production, and are easy to digest. They will make you feel full and will help you overcome your hunger. Now you're on the way to a good nights sleep.

Our body, in an effort to regulate the circadian cycle and to help us sleep, releases another powerful sleep aid called **Melatonin.**

Melatonin is synthesized in steps, first you consume the dietary amino acid called **tryptophan**, then as tryptophan is metabolized **serotonin** is produced, which proceeds the release of melatonin receptors, and last but not least the secretion of melatonin into the blood stream from pineal gland in the brain. The body completes this cycle after the sun goes down.

Melatonin is a hormone made in the pineal gland of the brain, produced naturally by plants and animals alike. It regulates our circadian rhythms, sleep, and wake cycles. Besides being a powerful sleep aid, another little known fact about the hormone melatonin is that it is also a predatory antioxidant that scavengers for toxins to be removed from our blood system.

Like all hormones, Melatonin levels are found to decline with age. Scientists conclude that some age related disorders may be due to the lack of this vital hormone.

This decline may be a factor in the growing rate of Alzheimer's disease, glucose intolerance (a precursor to type 2 diabetes), a compromised immune system, and cancer. Melatonin can be purchased at any drug store and can be taken every night to aid in falling asleep.

In studies done on rats and mice, the introduction of melatonin was found to increase their life-span by about 20%. Maybe because they were finally able to get a good nights sleep!

Are you Getting Any Loving?

We are all created as sexual beings. This energy center is called the sacral chakra, found below navel and the pubic area. It dominates our sexual desires, sexual sensations, and reproductive function as well. When this energy center is vibrating it will keep you from sleeping.

This is a powerful chakra's energy center that's also known as the "Qi" or "chi's" in the Chinese tradition or "prana" in the Sanskrit Indian tradition, meaning the vital life force. It usually expresses itself in the desire to make babies, guaranteeing the continuation of our species. After WWII when the men came home from war the life-force kicked in and we have now what is known as the Baby Boom of the 1950s.

When you comprehend the power of this chakra you see it can keep you awake until it is released.

The energy that is stored here in the form of sexual desire is always vibrating to some degree. When you are in a state of sexual desire your body will either, keep you awake until the energy is released, or eventually you will fall asleep exhausted . . .

The best way to release this energy is with the help of the partner of your choice. Releasing this energy will allow sleep to come next.

In case you are alone, you may have selected a celibate life and you planned your life this way. Most singles are unwilling participants who did not make the choice to live this lifestyle. Instead, more likely you are alone due to divorce, death of a loved one or other circumstances.

Sometimes just being alone is reason enough for you to have a hard time falling asleep.

If you are single you may have to find other means to release the energy, though rigorous exercise or some other way. Your personal decision to get a good night sleep sometimes depends on the release of this energy.

Right after the release of sexual energy your whole body settles into a relaxed state. The results are meant to release that pent up life-force energy from the sacral chakra. Sleep once again becomes possible.

Are you lonely?

In the age of computers with social media and instant connections online, we ask, who needs intimacy anymore. If you are having a relationship with your computer and not physically socializing with real people you can be counted among the many thousands.

The first thing you do when you wake in the morning is to turn on the computer and go to your E-Mail or social media account. Busy days, no time, full schedules, relationships are too much work, so the computer has become our new connection with the outside world. And we couldn't live without it.

Loneliness will keep you awake. If you want to get back to a regular sleep pattern you need to take the time to build relationships with real people . . . because; human intimacy is a gift and should be cherished. Our soul yearns to touch and be touched. Your computer is not your lover, your companion, nor your friend that you can depend on in times of need.

With the popularity of social media our computers fill the need to feel connected to the outside world. You know, it keeps you awake.

The experience of loneliness is a strong negative emotion that creates similar energy around the heart chakras. To change that energy you have to take positive steps. Join a club, a real estate club, a hiking club, a book club or travel club if that is your interest. Learn to dance, or learn a sport where you are meeting new people. Join an online dating service. Take some educational courses at the local college. Learn a new language. Join a church, synagogue, or spiritual affiliation of like minded people.

Step out from that experience of doing everything alone and make contact by phone or e-mail, but make contact. You may have to step out of your comfort zone to be the first one who reaches out to make contact, but just do it. When we take the risk and open ourselves up to another human being we change that experience. With your planned outreach effort, who knows you may meet your soul mate. Loneliness is a sleep robber.

By taking positive steps toward changing your circumstances, the negative vibes you are admitting, the feelings of loneliness, has now been transformed into positive intentions. You will sleep deeply when your heart is satisfied and your emotions turn to anticipation of meeting new people. Positive intentions (cause) will create positive results (effect).

We are not meant to be alone, but being alone does not have to equal loneliness.

There are times in our life when we will be alone. It may be by choice or it may be by the circumstances. It's OK if there is a period of grieving to overcome your sense of loss, but in time, this will change too. Whatever the occasion the heart chakra is super sensitive and has to be cleansed of past hurts, betrayal, lack of forgiveness and guilt. Here's how . . .

We all have this innate ability to visualize things in our mind and to do this we utilize a facility called our *minds eye.* Ephesians 1:18, May the eyes of your mind be enlightened.

With this eye we can visualize all sorts of things, from daydreams to fantasies, things that really do exist and things we imagine. It can be in the form of a snapshot or as vivid as if you were watching a movie on the big screen.

Visualization may seem strange at first, and using your mind's eye to perfect this facility takes practice, but developing this facility will be rewarding.

The way athletes are trained to win, is by using this technique called visualization. They're asked to picture themselves winning their sport first in their minds. Our brain does not discriminate whether this visualization is the real thing or not. The brain will automatically complete the game as they practiced in the mind, to win. So now we will use our power to visualize as a means to change our mind . . .

Ritual #1 Put the Garbage Out

Sit in a comfortable chair with your feet on the floor. First think of the negative emotions you are holding onto. Some of them may be sadness, grief, loneliness, unforgiveness, hate, fear, anger to name a few.

Using your **minds eye**, picture yourself depositing any negative emotions you are experiencing, (name them out loud) in a large see-thru garbage pail.

Think hard, and give a name to any and all negative emotions. You can see the level of the negative emotions in the clear see-thru pail. Fill it up . . .

After you finish stuffing them all in the large clear pail, see yourself putting the cover on and sealing it down tight. Then, put the garbage pail outside to be carted away by the garbage truck. Don't forget to actually see the garbage man in your mind, emptying your large pail into his truck and driving away. Repeat as often as needed.

Now to complete this ritual, make a conscious effort *to replace* those negative emotions that have been keeping you awake with an abundance of loving, joyful feelings. See yourself being surrounded by the love of a partner, lover, parent, or best friend celebrating your birthday! Actually feel the love!

True, results may take time and practice, but use it as an opportunity for growth.

If you are alone, it offers you the time to work on yourself with no one to distract you.

It will raise your consciousness to the next level. "Know Thyself." Take the time to examine who you are, what makes you tick, what ticks you off. Ask yourself these questions and write it down to remind yourself. Ask your friends to give you an assessment of you. Whatever is keeping you awake on this journey of life will surprise you when you just slow down to take notice . . .

Chapter 2

The Setting

W hen you experience sleep interruptions it may be due to the fact that your need for the same amount of sleep has changed.

Our need for sleep is not always consistent through-out our lives. Do not be alarmed if you always slept eight hours a night and now you only sleep five or six hours. As our body's age and transition to a different vibration our sleep patterns might be affected. On the other hand, some people just don't need eight hours of sleep at night. It may be temporary, due to stress or other factors. Sometimes you should allow these changes and just go with it. You only have three options to getting a good night sleep. First option, you can fall asleep naturally, lucky you. Second option, you can take a sleeping aid or alcohol to help you sleep. Third option, you can get creative by changing your environment, as presented in this short book.

Our daily activities or what we chose to do for our livelihood is known as our *Dharma*. This is the same as your purpose in life. It is what gives you the energy during the day to work. Whether in the form of a job or other forms of activities it may just be what you do. Even when tiredness reminds you through-out the day the body just can't stop. You can feel this energy. It wants to express itself through you. Your mind conceives it, then your body receives the energy to manifest it and you allow it to express. Wa-La, Creation.

As you express this energy, you are in the process of using it. Once used in expressing your purpose, (*Dharma*) the energy is discarded naturally, but more often, we bring our jobs into the bedroom at night.

The ritual below is one method to lower your current energy level. If you are in a high energy frequency job during the day at work, the first step to prepare for sleep is to lower that frequency.

The "act as if" technique is one powerful way to train your mind and lower your high energy frequency.

For example, before you go to bed at night stop thinking about the today's work day. Instead "act as if" tomorrow when you go to work, the boss will recognize your efforts, and you will receive an award.

To dissolve yesterday's worries "*act as if*" you have been doing that job successfully for years and it has been effortless and rewarding.

Refer to the "*act as if*" technique to overcome a high frequency career, that keep you worrying through-out the night. Another Ritual . . .

Ritual #2 Lower Your Frequency

Sit in a comfortable straight back chair with feet on the floor. Close your eyes and with the mind's eye see a wall in the middle of a big room. There is a light switch on that wall. Even though you are sitting, see yourself going over to the wall and dim the light slowly. Again, seeing with your minds eye and using your imagination, you can easily dim the switch slowly, slowly.

Your energy level and frequency will determine the brightness of the light. The higher your energy level, determines your frequency, and the brighter your light.

As you picture yourself lowering the switch, become aware of how you feel.

As you lower the switch and the light gets dimmer, your high energy frequency is slowly lowering and you begin to feel tired.

As you see yourself dimming the switch, see the light slowly dimming too. Then experience, (feel it) your body's vibration slowly moving to a lower frequency as the light dims.

Using your minds eye, visualization will help you manually switch that frenetic energy completely off.

If you don't physically feel it, then, "act as if" you do, and keep repeating the exercise, until you do.

When you prepare the mind, you offer your body a welcome place to the sleep.

Prepare and again prepare, because, for some of us precious sleep does not come easily. In this case, falling asleep must become a creative effort.

Sound Therapy

It's called sound therapy because sound is therapeutic. With the help of sound you may want to create rituals to help you fall asleep.

A ritual is a custom that is repeated over and over again and easy for your brain to retain. Mentioned in chapter 1 the bedroom is the place where you go to sleep and if you have a partner to share intimacy. Tune out the sounds of your day.

The bedroom is not the place to watch TV or work in the home/office on the computer. That kind of noise will tell the brain you are still in work mode. The work energy, (your dharma) you used during the day must come to a close.

It is said that music calms the wild beast. The fact that music has an enormous effect on our state of our mind cannot be stressed enough.

Sounds are also extremely effective when we listen to them to change our mood and make us feel differently. A recent study has concluded that the sounds of ocean waves have lowered blood pressure, hypertension, and relaxed elderly patients. Music or at least sounds should be an integral part of the process to help you sleep.

Sound and the vibration of sound are not only detected with the sense of hearing, but with the sense of its energy frequency experienced through our extra sensory perception.

Bi-Lineal beats and subliminal messages is the latest trend to help us find relaxation. Before you fall asleep the conscious self enters into an alpha frequency. In this state, the mind is prepared to receive those bi-lineal beats and subliminal messages.

It works well to help you sleep, when repeated for a minimum of thirty days without interruption.

If you are a visual person then watching Mp3s and seeing the hidden messages along with background sounds will help your subconscious mind prepare you to sleep.

The selection of the music or just sounds that you chose to lower your work day vibrations should be peaceful and quiet. Your choices of music should sooth your soul and bring joy to your heart chakras. Playing soft music before you sleep will put you in the mood to retire.

Aromatherapy

Our sense of smell is surely undervalued. With the exception of the sense of smell, all sensory input such as taste, touch, sight, hearing, and balance is sent to the thalamus part of the brain before being sent to the cerebral cortex.

Smell, more so than any other sense, is closely linked to parts of the brain that *process emotion and memory.*

Even though we assume smell is one of the basic senses, scientists are still discovering how we pick up odors, process them, and interpret them as smells. This is why researchers, perfume developers, and even government agencies are so interested about the sense of smell. We carry different receptors for different smells. We make associations from smells and now it's known that our memory plays a big role in those associations.

Since we will remember and recognize smells through the sense of smell, the use of aromas, scents, oils, and incense can stimulate our sense of smell to create a mood, an association to a good memory or a positive emotion.

For instance, the aroma of coffee brewing may suggest to the brain it's morning and time to get up and ready for work. So why can't you also create the mood using aroma's that are conducive to falling asleep. It may be the smell of your body after a long shower, the smell of the ocean or the smell of freshly washed clean sheets on the bed. Even the scent of a new born baby has helped some women to fall asleep. By stimulating the sense of smell you can joggle a good memory from the past that may help you fall sleep. Like the smell of your mother baking something in the oven or the smell of the night before Christmas.

Today there are a multitude of plug-in aromas, perfumes, and scents, specially created for freshening the air, romance, seduction, and why not sleeping. You can test a desired aroma that creates a mood and see if it helps you fall asleep.

The scent of Lavender has been known for centuries to create a relaxed mood.

You might combine the use of sound and aroma therapy to achieve falling asleep.

There are many products other than using candles for aromas in a closed bedroom. The burning of paraffin wax or incense gives off fumes that may promote an allergic reaction. More importantly, this may be a fire hazard when you do fall asleep.

Lighting

Before getting into bed, get into the habit of closing the shades or curtains to allow only interior lighting while you are still awake. The bedroom should have the capacity to be dark. The brain notices light and it could activate our biological clock, our circadian rhythm. Dimmers are necessary in the bedroom.

When experimenting with light therapy, a team of researchers at Thomas Jefferson Medical University, facilitated by Dr. George Brainard, identified a receptor in the human eye. They discovered that this receptor reacted to light, which in turn triggered the brain to suppress the production of melatonin. This research revealed that **light is responsible** for our bodies lack of melatonin production when needed and disrupting our natural circadian rhythms.

For the sake of a good night sleep, create your bedroom to be a tranquil and a meditative environment.

The use of deep tones and mellow colors will create a relaxing environment. As discussed for sleeping, it is essential the room be completely dark and the shades or curtains closed.

However, some people need to keep a night light on to feel safe. Whatever your preference is, it is paramount that the room is dark; there is a sense of privacy and a feeling of security in the room.

If the computer is in your bedroom it should be turned completely off. The computer screen is filled with exciting images that are designed and marketed to grab our attention. It's impossible to fall asleep under these circumstances. Our computers give off electromagnetic vibrations and the flashing of computer lights will disrupt your need to sleep.

Turn off all technology except a sound machine if you use one.

The uses of colored light bulbs that can be dimmed are a neat way to create the mood. Decorative night lights and sconce lighting can display soft shadows that give a feeling of comfort. Using candles for lighting effects in the bedroom is unsafe for obvious reasons. The aroma alone can be overpowering in a small closed off room.

The Right Temperature

The temperature has to be just right too. No joke, you won't fall asleep if it's too hot, or too cold, so be aware of your surroundings.

If you live in a colder climate and it happens to be winter, you may feel chilled to the bone. During these cold winter nights, take a warm bath before bedtime. This will bring your body temperature back to normal. There is something to be said about warm water encompassing your entire body.

Is it a reminder of our mother's womb that helps us relax this deeply?

If you prefer a shower, this is fine too. Just stand in the water for a few minutes until you feel your body temperature change. Sleep becomes effortless when your body is comfortable in its own skin.

Again, not too hot and not too cold, but the water temperature should be just right. Try to bring your body's temperature to a place where you feel thoroughly relaxed.

It may seem un-important, but two degrees can make a difference whether or not you can fall asleep. If you live in the tropics and need the air conditioner on to fall asleep, better turn it down to that sleeping temperature or you might be awake to see the sunrise.

Be aware of the fresh oxygen in the room that is available. When you have all the widows closed the temperature can warm up overnight. Turn your fan on low to keep the oxygen flowing around the room.

Now that you've created the setting, you are almost ready to turn off the switch. Read again chapter two, **ritual #2** and learn how to successfully turn off your switch.

Chapter 3

The Energy Centers

Both the Western and Eastern philosophies recognized that we as human beings are made up of two bodies. These two bodies are known as the physical body which can be seen and the spirit or etheric body which is invisible.

Technology has advanced so much with the use of **Kirlian photography;** we are now able to see the second body. This spirit or etheric body that is now visible with the help of this special photography, is known as the *Aura*. It expresses itself as **the halo of energy** that surrounds you.

Our Aura that we can now see is also referred to as our bio-energy field. It looks like a blueprint of our physical body.

It is a highly charged electro-magnetic field surrounding our bodies with color and light vibrating at high frequencies. It is believed that this energy continues, even after our bodies cease to exist.

In this last decade we've learned through Quantum Physics, that everything is energy.

Our bodies were created with receptors to receive this energy. The body consists of the seven chakras. The seven chakras act as receptors that are also warehouses to store and distribute the energy it receives.

Chakra is an Indian word meaning motion and is shaped like a wheel. In other words our chakras or the wheels are spinning with energy. As I noted before and you will hear through-out this book, the Chakras are the body's energy centers and when blocked can lead to insomnia.

The Chinese became aware centuries ago of how energy flows through the body. Their knowledge of "blocked energy" has given birth to the ancient practice of acupuncture.

With our new understanding of how the brain works we can use the powerful techniques in this book to accomplish a good night sleep.

This book explains how stored energy can be stuck energy and keep us from falling asleep.

Tossing & Turning

Remember those long nights, and even though the body is comfortable in the new bed you just bought, you can not stop doing it. You can't stop tossing and turning.

When your body starts this kind of movement, it is time to take action. If you wait to see if the tossing and turning will cease, you are wasting time. Get out of the bed and take a warm shower, bath or do some yoga stretching exercise.

Meditation is almost impossible during this phase of insomnia. There is need for action, movement, stretching, or some form of exercise.

The only way to disrupt the cycle of tossing and turning is to physically change the rhythm of your body's movements. If not, when you look at the clock again you will see hours have passed and you're still tossing and turning.

When we toss and turn it is a sign that our body is trying to release pent up energy. Energy that is blocked, hasn't been distributed properly, or has yet to be released naturally. The tossing and turning cycle is one way that your body will try to eliminate that un-used energy.

Unfortunately this cycle can last for hours, unless you work off the excess energy or until finally you are exhausted and fall asleep.

What else can an insomniac do with all their energy, but toss and turn?

Hey, bet you thought you were tired.

This is true, you are tired, but this may be the very reason you are holding onto the energy, because you are tired. Now it's impossible to sleep because you have all this pent up energy that you're holding onto. It turns into a vicious cycle.

The Spinning Record

We have all had the experience of taking our problems to bed with us. Our mind will think about whatever problems challenged us during the day and this repeats over and over like a spinning record.

These thoughts are congested or blocked energy. Our thinking becomes jumbled and like other problems we solve regularly, these problems evade solutions. This is recognized as stress.

We all respond to stress and it is necessary to our survival, called fight or flight. The problem is without stress we would not be able to act in times of danger. Many people say they perform best under some stress. Other people are immobilized by the fear stress creates, like a deer in headlights.

The signs of stress are tight muscles, clenching or grinding your teeth, breathing rapidly and sweating profusely. Different people have many different responses to stress. The energy you release while you respond to stress is either physical or mental, so either your body will toss and turn or your thoughts spin like a broken record and you will not be able to sleep.

The first step is to recognize what is happening in your body, mind and spirit.

To solve your toss and turn or spinning record sleepless nights, sit up in bed immediately, turn on the lamp, and reach for your pen and paper you keep near the bed. Now, record exactly what your thoughts are telling you.

First, you must become aware that there is a problem.

Second, there is a group of problems that are disrupting your sleep because they are ready to be solved.

It's easy to see that our mind is presenting them to us, in an effort to remind us to write them down, *now*. If you do fall asleep you may forget the problem in the morning, but that night you are kept awake again. Our mind keeps us awake until we take charge of the situation; otherwise the problems will keep spinning round like a broken record.

By writing it down the problem is visibly on paper so that it becomes clear. In the morning you can refer to it when it's ready to be solved. As soon as you transferred the problem to paper ask your brain to bring you the necessary solution in your dreams that night.

The purpose of this exercise is first to release the energy by writing the problem on paper and second, solve it later so you can sleep tonight.

When they are arranged in order on paper, your mind can let go of that energy. Set it on the table next to the bed authorizing your subconscious mind to work on the solutions in your dreams.

It is important that you verbalize *this instruction* to your mind. Let your dreams come up with the best solution to your problem, while you are asleep. When you instruct your mind, the solutions will begin to surface from your subconscious to your conscious mind. Be aware of your dreams, because the solution that will help you sleep can come in this form.

Where does the energy come from?

The reason I write about energy, is so that you understand the basics and that energy can affect your sleep or lack thereof.

Since the Industrial revolution, we began our mad consumption of electricity and oil. Since the explosion of the technological revolution, almost everyone who owns a computer, cell phone, or electronic communication device leaves it plugged in 24 hours a day.

As human beings we have also increased our dependence on a limitless energy that powers our bodies and gives us life.

Some energy comes from an earthly source like the sun, earth, or wind. Some energy comes from earth's bounty as the food we eat. Then, some energy is manufactured from our own bodies, and some energy is pure energy that comes from a mysterious source.

Some people call it God, the creator, their higher power or their source. Acts 17:28 *It is in God we live and move, and have my being*

In the 21st century our need for the energy that comes from outside our being has expanded exponentially. Our daily activities that require us to multi-task and utilize electronic equipment grows everyday. Operating computers, cell phones, smart phones, e-mail, Ipads, and social media networks have opened up new electromagnetic frequencies of energy bombarding us continuously.

Not only do we overeat when we are tired, trying to produce more energy, we lose sleep in an effort to hold onto energy when we are tired.

Could our body, mind and spirit live without that unlimited, invisible thing we call energy?

With the use of these electronic tools to communicate and interact with each other, our bodies are transferring energy to the chakras at a velocity unlike anything similar in the history of mankind.

The other source of energy, which has a profound effect on our own energy level, is our interaction with other people or lack of contact with others, which effect our emotions.

Emotions are energy, powerful energy that can empower you or deflate you. When emotional energy is plugged into the wrong outlet it will rob you of sleep.

Emotional pain taught me a valuable lesson. An example of my own self discovery is when during an argument with my partner; I noticed how much negative energy was exchanged during these battles. After one of these battles my body was vibrating with all this energy, I could feel my chakras spinning, but still I couldn't let it go . . . I tossed and turned that night until I knew I wouldn't sleep a wink. After my self examination the cause became clear that I was responsible for creating the negative energy.

The emotional pain which turned into negative energy would not let me sleep.

I acknowledged my part and asked my partner if we can make up.

When we forgave each other, I realized by letting go of the hostility, it released the negative energy. After that, we both softened up and finally fell asleep.

The practice of the rituals in this book will help you gain control over your negative emotions and the energy it creates that keeps you from falling asleep.

The energy that comes from our emotions can either run our life or ruin our life.

Put in simple terms; negative emotional energy is a resource that continues supplying the fuel for your insomnia.

Then, there is bad emotions (energy) that are inflicted upon us from other people. Emotions or feelings, good or bad, cause a memory. Negative memories if stored (not forgiven) are trapped emotional energy in our energy warehouse, the chakras.

We cannot always control emotional pain, who or what caused it, but we can control our reaction to it. Clearing the conscience feels as good as, climbing into a freshly made bed with warm clean sheets, right after bathing. With a clear conscience you succumb to falling asleep easily and effortlessly.

We can't see energy but we know it exists. We can't see electricity either, but it powers everything we do. We are constantly receiving energy in huge quantities as much or more than the air we breathe, it's always there.

After use, energy is usually discharged automatically. When we experience pain in our back, neck or any area of the body that may indicate trapped energy is there.

Chapter 4

Pain Keeps You Awake

P ain is a very complicated part of our body's makeup. Really, what is the purpose of pain and where does it come from?

It can come from a physical, emotional, spiritual or an undefined source.

Pain is a major cause for the lack of sleep.

It's impossible to fall asleep when you have constant pain, without the use of drugs. Chronic pain of any kind will bring about big changes in your sleep patterns.

Likewise, this may be the other purpose for pain, not to keep you awake, but to cause change in your life. Maybe it's there to inform us that we are holding onto past hurts and remain unforgiving. The pain that keeps you awake is a message that needs to be examined.

Some pain cannot be identified. It's there and it hurts, but it eludes you. Undefined pain may be the result of our guilt-ridden world.

To Forgive is Divine

This is a biggy, after being tried and tested by experience, is one of the reasons we may find it hard to sleep. That may be why it says in the bible, never let the sun go down on your anger . . . Ephesians 4:26

Your emotions might still be tied up with past hurts. That someone broke your heart, cheated on you, abandoned you, or wrongfully accused you; make's it hard to forgive. When faced with countless painful and unfortunate relationships through-out our lives, holding onto those left over emotions will likely keep you earthbound (stuck) and unhappy.

Being able to forgive might be the hardest thing you have ever done, or the bravest, but it will expand your soul.

Even after you have forgiven others, guilt will not let you sleep, unless you forgive yourself.

The ritual I use to rid myself of the past un-forgiveness and guilt is:

Ritual #3 Release and Ship Out

Sit in a comfortable chair in a quiet place, where you can have privacy.

Gather up all the bad feelings you have about yourself, including guilt, shame, envy, anger, hate, and fear. Especially the guilt you wear around your neck, because you think you aren't doing enough for your parents, children, spouse, friends, others. This might take a few minutes . . .

Put all these feeling in a clear garbage bag so you can take it with you . . .

In your mind's eye see yourself going to the river where you will find a big blue sail boat.

Empty the clear garbage bag and fill the boat with all the bad feelings you were able to recover and launch it out to sea.

Watch as the boat finally disappears from sight. At the same time *repeat in your mind that you release* all those bad feelings that you emptied on the boat, then *invite and receive* the flow of your creative energy.

With the release and then disappearance of the boat, likely the bad feelings will change. Claim that they are far and gone out to sea. They no longer make you feel anything, because you barely remember what caused them.

A guilt free sleep comes easily to those who can forgive themselves and others.

When we hold onto guilt it traps energy. Many of us are in a state of constant self criticism before we realize it. We are not aware of these unconscious feelings, but they probably began with our parents, teachers, and our own erroneous beliefs.

Guilt plays an important role in our sense of self. Guilt stops positive energy from expressing. It is hard to impossible to release this blocked energy without becoming aware of the reason WHY the guilt exists in the first place. When self discovery leads you to the reason for your guilt, you can forgive yourself and finally fall asleep.

Spiritual Restoration

This is so subtle that it often goes undetected as one of the reasons we haven't been able to fall sleep.

We have all experienced sleepless nights during times of great stress, when life's problems seem to overwhelm us.

During these times, sleep, may not be easily found, but there is hope.

There is a remedy to resolve those deep dark feelings of self doubt and despair.

It's an age old practice that is just as popular today as ever and that is called prayer.

Prayer substantiates faith, which creates a connection to your higher power. That means, when you pray, you acknowledge that you believe God hears the prayer . . .

When you make this connection a light will begin to shine on the darkness that surrounds you.

Focused prayer, like meditation can be successful at helping you sleep.

It's a fact that it alters your consciousness to rest in the alpha state and it also lowers your (frequency) vibration.

Best of all, you have now become conscious and made the connection that your higher power is there. Through the act of prayer, *you can act as if,* you are really in a relationship with your higher power.

There is no longer any reason to feel alone when life's problems try to overwhelm you.

Chapter 5

Yawning and Stretching

Humans are not the only animals that yawn, many living creatures, such as cats, dogs and fish do. A human fetus has been observed yawning in their mother's womb. Everyone knows that yawning is contagious. As soon as we see someone else yawn there is an involuntary action, an automatic reflex that kicks in, which causes us to yawn. What's that?

Scientists have no clue, but have been theorizing for years and still cannot explain, why we yawn?

I don't pretend to be smarter than a scientist, but this I do know; we all have had a good yawn at some point in our lives when we are tired.

Could be, another reason why we yawn is that our body is discarding pent up energy . . . .

Yes but, scientists want to know, exactly, what purpose does yawning serve? Once we experience a good yawn and this energy is discarded, our bodies can feel tired, bored, or very relaxed and will start tuning out. Is it possible that yawning also acts as a signal to the brain to slow the body down and fall asleep?

You can feel the satisfactory relief after a good yawn. It stretches the facial muscles and at the same time relaxes them as we open our mouth wide. We inhale a deep breathe of oxygen and exhale carbon dioxide along with pent up energy. Sometimes a deep guttural sound will accompany it to give us more relief.

The risorius muscles that are connected to the jaw at the temporomandibular joint (a small joint located in front of the ear where the skull and lower jaw meet) are also connected to the base of the brain. So that a good yawn is signaling the brain instantly. The brain also creates neurotransmitters that are sent out that can generate yawning. Could it be that the message (it's time for sleep) is being sent through-out the body.

In this chapter, a new ritual to try is the practice of yawning and stretching the jaw to send a signal to the brain.

Remember to instruct the brain (verbally) often, that every time you yawn, it will be the signal that slows down your metabolism. You're body needs rest and you want to be able to fall sleep tonight.

Ritual #4 Yawning Your Way to Sleep

Stretch your arms over your head, and then stretch your arms back behind your head. Clasp your hands together, but continue to hold them up over your head. Release those tense muscles before you lay in bed. Stretch your limbs out by extending them out as far as you can.

Even if you do not feel like yawning at the moment, act as if you do. Open your mouth wide and extend the lower jaw as if you were popping your clogged ears. Try yawning now. If this didn't turn into a real yawn keep trying, until it does. You can continue to practice this until you have really yawned four or more times or until tiredness follows.

When I use this method and stretch, I yawn every time and will yawn many times after that.

If you can't yawn then watch a video tape on youtube. com of people yawning. Yawning is contagious. Maybe it will help us send that signal to the brain that we are tired and ready to fall sleep.

Holistic vs. Drugs

Since the 60s many USA citizens have become dependent on drugs to help them sleep. These drugs mask our sleep problem rather than understand the nature of them. We all have resorted to drugs to get to sleep when sleep eludes us. If not we might be up all night, so we take action and quickly go for the drugs to get the sleep we need.

I too have walked down this road and chosen the quick fix. The problem is that after frequent use we develop a resistance to the drugs and have to take larger quantities to get the sleep we need. Finally, when we wake up in the morning we're in a fog for hours afterwards.

Now we're faced with a new set of problems, we have developed a dependency on drugs to help us sleep. Guilt follows as we blame ourselves for allowing this to happen.

After you give up the drugs, it may take awhile to get back to the place were you can fall asleep naturally.

Living at the end of the twentieth century we've re-discovered natural remedies passed down from our ancestors to help us sleep.

The powers of natural herbs have demonstrated they can successfully bring on sleep; have few side effects and no dependency issues. Melatonin is just one over the counter, natural, non-narcotic, and non habit forming sleep aid that works, and therefore is safe to take daily.

Always consult your primary physician before taking any natural supplements.

Teas to Help You Sleep

In this chapter we will address the use of teas as a temporary aid to help bring on sleep. From experience I can assure you, if the teas are prepared as directed you will get results. The blending of herbs, roots, and leaves has created formulas that will send you into a deep sleep if you drink it before bedtime.

Look for natural herbs made into teas that can restore sleep. Chamomile, Valerian root, lavender, and Jarrow to name a few. Stay away from caffeinated teas.

Whether you decide to use foods, vitamins, natural supplements, herbs, or teas, all are created by nature for the very purpose to help you sleep.

Getting enough sleep each night is crucial for the repair and replication of healthy cells.

Every night while we sleep our liver goes through a cleaning and flushing process to remove toxins, dead cells, and debris in the blood.

This is an automatic process by our body to cleanse it and keep it healthy.

Every night, before we close our eyes to sleep, we should make it a habit until it becomes automatic, to cleanse our heart and mind from the stress of the day.

Then as we sleep the stagnant energy and bad vibes that we picked up during our waking time are flushed out.

Getting a good night sleep is the purpose of this little book.

I hope by sharing some of my tried and true methods and intentional rituals you can discover how to find the way for sleep to return.

GOODNIGHT